Fruits : The Ultimate Cure

Table of Contents

I. Introduction

A. Definition of Fruit

Fruits are an integral part of our diet and have been for thousands of years. They are sweet, juicy, and come in a wide variety of colors and flavors. However, what exactly is a fruit? The definition of fruits can vary depending on who you ask, but generally, it refers to the edible part of a plant that contains seeds.

To be more specific, a fruit is the mature ovary of a flowering plant. When the flower is pollinated, the ovary begins to grow and develop into a fruit. The purpose of the fruit is to protect and nourish the seeds until they are ready to be dispersed.

Fruits come in many different shapes and sizes. Some are small, like blueberries, while others can grow to be quite large, like watermelons. They can be round, oblong, or even heart-shaped. They can be eaten raw or cooked and can be used in a variety of dishes, from sweet to savory.

Fruits are also a good source of nutrients. They are high in vitamins, minerals, and fiber, and are generally low in calories. They can help lower the risk of chronic diseases, such as heart disease, cancer, and diabetes. Eating a variety of fruits can help maintain a healthy diet and provide the necessary nutrients the body needs.

However, there are some fruits that are commonly mistaken for vegetables. For example, tomatoes are often thought of as a vegetable, but they are actually a fruit. This is because they develop from the ovary of a flower and contain seeds.

Similarly, avocados are often thought of as vegetables, but they are also a fruit. They develop from a flower and contain a seed. This can be confusing, but it is important to remember that fruits are defined by their reproductive structure, not by their taste or culinary use.

In conclusion, fruits are an essential part of a healthy diet. They are defined as the mature ovary of a flowering plant and come in a variety of shapes and sizes. They are high in nutrients and can help lower the risk of chronic diseases. While some fruits are commonly mistaken for vegetables, it is important to remember that fruits are defined by their reproductive structure. So the next time you enjoy a juicy apple or a refreshing slice of watermelon, remember that you are not just indulging in a delicious treat, but also nourishing your body with important nutrients.

B. Importance of fruits in our diet

Fruits are an essential part of a healthy diet. They provide us with essential nutrients that help us maintain good health and prevent diseases. A diet that includes a variety of fruits can help you meet your daily nutritional requirements while also satisfying your taste buds.
Here are some reasons why fruits are important in our diet:
Provide essential vitamins and minerals

1. Fruits are an excellent source of vitamins and minerals, which are essential for our overall health. They are rich in vitamin C, vitamin A, potassium, and folate, which are necessary for healthy skin, bones, and teeth. Fruits like oranges, kiwis, and strawberries are rich in vitamin C, while bananas and avocados are rich in potassium.

Boost immune system

2. Fruits are packed with antioxidants, which are known to boost the immune system. These antioxidants help to fight off harmful free radicals that can damage our cells and lead to chronic diseases like cancer and heart disease. Fruits like berries, citrus fruits, and melons are particularly high in antioxidants.

Improve digestion

3. Fruits are a good source of dietary fiber, which helps to improve digestion and prevent constipation. Fiber also helps to lower cholesterol levels and reduce the risk of heart disease. Fruits like apples, pears, and berries are particularly high in fiber.

Aid weight loss

4. Fruits are low in calories and high in fiber, making them an excellent food for weight loss. They can help to reduce hunger

and prevent overeating. Fruits like apples, oranges, and grapes are particularly good for weight loss.

Promote heart health

5. Fruits are rich in potassium, which is known to lower blood pressure and reduce the risk of heart disease. They are also low in saturated fat and cholesterol, making them a heart-healthy food. Fruits like pomegranates, blueberries, and strawberries are particularly good for heart health.

In conclusion, fruits are an essential part of a healthy diet. They provide us with essential vitamins, minerals, and fiber, which help us maintain good health and prevent diseases. Eating a variety of fruits can help you meet your daily nutritional requirements while also satisfying your taste buds. So, make sure to include a variety of fruits in your daily diet for good health.

C. Nutritional value of fruits

Fruits are an excellent source of essential nutrients that are vital for the healthy functioning of the human body. They are rich in vitamins, minerals, fiber, and antioxidants, which provide a wide range of health benefits. In this article, we will discuss the nutritional value of fruits and why they should be a part of a healthy diet.

Vitamins and Minerals

Fruits are a great source of vitamins and minerals that are necessary for maintaining optimal health. They contain high levels of vitamin C, vitamin A, folate, and potassium, among others. Vitamin C is essential for the growth and repair of tissues in the body, while vitamin A is crucial for maintaining healthy vision and skin. Potassium is necessary for regulating blood pressure and preventing heart disease.

Fiber

Fruits are an excellent source of dietary fiber, which is important for maintaining healthy digestion and preventing constipation. Fiber helps to regulate bowel movements and reduces the risk of colon cancer. It also helps to control blood sugar levels and can reduce the risk of type 2 diabetes.

Antioxidants

Fruits are rich in antioxidants, which are important for protecting the body from damage caused by harmful free radicals. Free radicals can damage cells and contribute to the development of chronic diseases such as cancer and heart disease. Antioxidants help to neutralize these free radicals and protect the body from their harmful effects. Fruits such as blueberries, strawberries, and raspberries are particularly rich in antioxidants.

Low in Calories

Most fruits are low in calories, making them an excellent food for weight management. They are a great option for snacking between meals and can help to reduce hunger and prevent overeating. Fruits like apples, oranges, and grapes are low in calories and high in fiber, making them a great choice for those trying to lose weight.

Variety

There is a wide variety of fruits available, each with their unique nutritional benefits. For example, citrus fruits like oranges and grapefruits are high in vitamin C, while bananas and avocados are rich in potassium. Berries are an excellent source of antioxidants, and kiwi fruit is rich in vitamin K. By including a variety of fruits in your diet, you can ensure that you are getting a wide range of essential nutrients.

In conclusion, fruits are an excellent source of essential nutrients that are necessary for maintaining optimal health. They are rich in vitamins, minerals, fiber, and antioxidants, among others. By including a variety of fruits in your diet, you can ensure that you are getting a wide range of essential nutrients that can provide a wide range of health benefits. So, make sure to include fruits in your daily diet for good health.

D. Purpose of the book

Eating fruits is an important part of maintaining a healthy and balanced diet. The purpose of eating fruits is to provide the body with essential nutrients that promote overall health and prevent chronic diseases. Fruits are rich in vitamins, minerals, antioxidants, and fiber, which provide numerous health benefits.

One of the primary purposes of eating fruits is to boost the immune system. Fruits are high in vitamin C, which helps strengthen the immune system and protect against infections and diseases. They also contain other vitamins and minerals such as vitamin A, vitamin E, and zinc, which support immune function and help the body fight off harmful pathogens.

Eating fruits can also help reduce the risk of chronic diseases such as cancer, heart disease, and diabetes. Fruits are rich in antioxidants, which help protect the body against cellular damage caused by free radicals. Free radicals are unstable molecules that can damage cells and contribute to the development of chronic diseases. Antioxidants neutralize free radicals and help prevent cellular damage.

Fruits are also an excellent source of dietary fiber, which promotes digestive health and helps prevent constipation. Fiber helps keep the digestive system running smoothly by adding bulk to stool and promoting regular bowel movements. Eating a diet rich in fiber can also help lower cholesterol levels and reduce the risk of heart disease.

Another purpose of eating fruits is to maintain a healthy weight. Fruits are low in calories and high in fiber, which can help reduce calorie intake and promote feelings of fullness. Eating fruits as part of a balanced diet can help prevent overeating and contribute to healthy weight management.

In addition to their nutritional benefits, eating fruits can also be a delicious and enjoyable experience. Fruits come in a wide variety of colors, flavors, and te

In conclusion, the purpose of eating fruits is to provide the body with essential nutrients that promote overall health and prevent chronic diseases. Fruits are an excellent source of vitamins, minerals, antioxidants, and fiber, which provide numerous health benefits. By incorporating fruits into a balanced diet, individuals can improve their health and enjoy a delicious and nutritious eating experience, making them a versatile ingredient in many different dishes. Incorporating fruits into meals and snacks can help add variety and flavor to a healthy diet.

II. History of Fruits

A. Origins and domestication of fruits

Fruits have been a part of the human diet for thousands of years, and their origins and domestication can be traced back to ancient times. The earliest evidence of fruit consumption comes from the fossil record, where seeds and other plant remains have been found at archaeological sites dating back to the Paleolithic era.

The process of fruit domestication began with early humans gathering and selecting wild fruits for consumption. Over time, humans began to cultivate and selectively breed fruits to produce desirable traits such as size, flavor, and texture. This process led to the development of new fruit varieties and the eventual domestication of many common fruits that we enjoy today.

One of the earliest fruits to be domesticated was the fig, which was cultivated in the Middle East and Mediterranean regions around 11,000 years ago. The date palm, another important fruit in the Middle East, was domesticated around 8,000 years ago. In Asia, rice and mango were domesticated around 4,000 years ago, while bananas were domesticated in Southeast Asia around 7,000 years ago.

In the Americas, several important fruits were domesticated by indigenous peoples. The avocado was domesticated in Mexico and Central America around 5,000 years ago, while the tomato was domesticated in South America around 2,500 years ago. Other important domesticated fruits in the Americas include strawberries, blueberries, and cranberries.

The process of fruit domestication was not limited to selective breeding. Humans also developed new methods of cultivation, such as grafting and hybridization, to produce new fruit varieties. Grafting involves joining together different parts of plants to create a new hybrid plant, while hybridization involves cross-breeding different plant varieties to produce new traits.

Today, fruits are an important part of the human diet and are grown and consumed around the world. Many of the fruits we enjoy today are the result of centuries of domestication and selective breeding. Fruits not only provide important nutritional benefits but also play an important role in cultural traditions and celebrations. Understanding the origins and domestication of fruits can help us appreciate their importance and significance in human history and culture.

B. Cultural significance of fruits

Fruits have played an important role in human culture throughout history, and their cultural significance can be seen in various aspects of society, including religion, art, literature, and cuisine. Fruits have been celebrated for their nutritional value, aesthetic beauty, and symbolism. In many cultures, fruits have religious significance. In Hinduism, for example, the banana tree is considered sacred and is associated with the goddess Lakshmi. In Christianity, the apple is often associated with the story of Adam and Eve in the Garden of Eden. The pomegranate is also considered a symbol of fertility and abundance in many cultures, and is often associated with the goddess Persephone in Greek mythology. Fruits have also been the subject of many works of art and literature. Paintings of fruit bowls, for example, have been popular since the Renaissance and were used to symbolize wealth and abundance. In literature, fruits have been used as symbols to represent different ideas or emotions. The apple, for example, has been used as a symbol of temptation, while the fig has been used as a symbol of sensuality.

Fruits also play an important role in cuisine and culinary traditions. Many cultures have specific dishes and recipes that feature fruits as a main ingredient. In Mediterranean cuisine, for example, figs and dates are often used in savory dishes, while pomegranates are used in salads and stews. In Thai cuisine, mangoes are used in both sweet and savory dishes, and are often paired with spicy flavors.

Fruits also play an important role in celebrations and festivals. In China, the Chinese New Year is celebrated with the tradition of offering oranges to friends and family as a symbol of good luck and prosperity. In Mexico, the Day of the Dead festival is celebrated with the tradition of creating elaborate altars that include offerings of fruit, including oranges, apples, and pomegranates.

In conclusion, fruits have a rich cultural significance and have played an important role in human history and society. Fruits have been celebrated for their nutritional value, aesthetic beauty, and symbolic meanings. Whether used in religion, art, literature, cuisine, or celebrations, fruits continue to be an important part of human culture and traditions.

C. Fruits in ancient civilizations

Fruits have been an important part of human civilization for thousands of years, and their use and significance can be traced back to ancient times. In many ancient civilizations, fruits played a significant role in the economy, religion, and daily life of people.

One of the earliest civilizations where fruits played a significant role was ancient Egypt. The Egyptians cultivated a variety of fruits, including grapes, figs, dates, and pomegranates. Fruits were not only an important source of nutrition but were also used for medicinal purposes and religious rituals. The pomegranate, in particular, was associated with fertility and was used in offerings to the gods.

In ancient Greece, fruits were also an important part of daily life. The Greeks cultivated a variety of fruits, including grapes, figs, and olives. Fruits were often used in religious rituals and were seen as symbols of wealth and abundance. In Greek mythology, the pomegranate was associated with the goddess Persephone, and its seeds were seen as a symbol of rebirth.

In ancient Rome, fruits were also an important part of daily life and were cultivated for both nutrition and trade. The Romans imported fruits from all over the Mediterranean, including figs, dates, and pomegranates. Fruits were often used in feasts and celebrations and were seen as a symbol of wealth and status. The apple, in particular, was associated with the goddess Venus and was seen as a symbol of love and beauty.

In ancient China, fruits were also an important part of daily life and were cultivated for both nutrition and medicinal purposes. The Chinese cultivated a variety of fruits, including peaches, plums, and apricots. Fruits were often used in traditional Chinese medicine and were believed to have healing properties. Fruits were also used in festivals and celebrations, including the Chinese New Year, where oranges were given as gifts as a symbol of good luck and prosperity.

In conclusion, fruits have played an important role in ancient civilizations, from Egypt to China. Fruits were not only an important source of nutrition but were also used for medicinal purposes, religious rituals, and celebrations. Fruits continue to be an important part of human culture and society today, and their significance and value can be traced back to the earliest civilizations in human history.

D. Historical uses of fruits

Fruits have been used by humans for various purposes throughout history, including as a source of nutrition, medicine, and religious significance. The historical uses of fruits are diverse and have evolved over time with changing cultural practices and scientific advancements.

One of the earliest historical uses of fruits was as a source of nutrition. Fruits were consumed by early humans as a source of essential vitamins and minerals, and as a way to supplement their diets. Fruits were also important in early agriculture and trade, with some fruits being highly prized and sought after, such as dates in ancient Egypt.

Fruits were also used for medicinal purposes in many cultures. In ancient Greece and Rome, fruits were used to treat a variety of ailments, including digestive issues, respiratory problems, and skin conditions. The Greek physician Hippocrates, known as the father of modern medicine, recommended fruits such as figs and grapes for their health benefits.

Religious significance was another historical use of fruits. In ancient Egypt, pomegranates were used in offerings to the gods and were associated with fertility. In Christianity, the apple was associated with the story of Adam and Eve and represented temptation and sin. In Hinduism, the banana tree is considered sacred and is associated with the goddess Lakshmi.

Fruits were also used for practical purposes throughout history. For example, the juice of the lemon was used by sailors to prevent scurvy during long sea voyages. The peel of the orange was used to make fragrances and cosmetics in ancient China and Rome.

In more recent history, fruits have been used in the food and beverage industry. The invention of the refrigerated railroad car in the late 1800s allowed for the transportation of fruits across long distances, leading to the development of the fruit canning and juice industries.

In conclusion, fruits have been used for a variety of purposes throughout history, including as a source of nutrition, medicine, and religious significance. Fruits have played an important role in human culture and society and continue to be an important part of our daily lives today. The historical uses of fruits have evolved over time with changing cultural practices and scientific advancements, and fruits remain a valuable and versatile resource.

III. Types of Fruits

A. Citrus fruits

Citrus fruits are a group of fruits that are known for their tangy, acidic flavor and high vitamin C content. The citrus fruit family includes well-known fruits such as oranges, lemons, limes, grapefruits, and tangerines. Citrus fruits are a popular choice for both eating and juicing, and they are also used in cooking, baking, and as a flavoring agent in a wide range of foods and drinks.

Citrus fruits are native to tropical and subtropical regions of Asia and are believed to have originated in the Himalayan foothills. From there, citrus fruits were introduced to the Mediterranean region, where they became an important part of the diet and culture. Today, citrus fruits are grown in many parts of the world, including the United States, Mexico, Brazil, Spain, and Italy.

Citrus fruits are not only delicious but also have numerous health benefits. They are high in vitamin C, which is important for immune system health and helps the body absorb iron. Citrus fruits also contain other essential vitamins and minerals, such as vitamin A, potassium, and folate. Some citrus fruits, such as grapefruits, are also a good source of dietary fiber.

In addition to their nutritional value, citrus fruits have also been found to have medicinal properties. For example, the flavonoids found in citrus fruits have been shown to have antioxidant properties, which can help protect against cancer and cardiovascular disease. Citrus fruits are also believed to have anti-inflammatory properties and can help lower cholesterol levels.

Citrus fruits have many culinary uses as well. Oranges and lemons are commonly used in baking and as a flavoring agent in dishes such as marinades and salad dressings. Limes are often used in cocktails and to add flavor to Mexican and Latin American dishes. Grapefruits are commonly eaten for breakfast, and tangerines make for a convenient and healthy snack.

In conclusion, citrus fruits are a delicious and nutritious group of fruits that have been enjoyed by humans for centuries. They are rich in vitamins and minerals, have numerous health benefits, and are a versatile ingredient in a wide range of foods and drinks. Whether eaten fresh, juiced, or used in cooking, citrus fruits are a delicious and healthy addition to any diet.

B. Berries

Berries are a group of small, colorful fruits that are known for their sweet and tangy flavor. The berry family includes popular fruits such as strawberries, blueberries, raspberries, blackberries, and cranberries. Berries are not only delicious but also have numerous health benefits, making them a popular choice for people looking to add more fruit to their diet.

Berries are native to many different parts of the world, including North America, Europe, and Asia. They grow on small shrubs or vines and are usually harvested by hand. Berries are a rich source of vitamins, minerals, and antioxidants, and they are low in calories and high in fiber.

One of the key health benefits of berries is their high antioxidant content. Antioxidants are compounds that help protect the body against damage from free radicals, which can contribute to the development of cancer and other diseases. Berries are particularly high in anthocyanins, a type of antioxidant that gives berries their bright color and has been shown to have anti-inflammatory and anticancer properties.

Berries are also a good source of vitamin C, which is important for immune system health and helps the body absorb iron. They are also high in dietary fiber, which can help regulate digestion and reduce the risk of heart disease and type 2 diabetes.

Berries are a versatile ingredient in a wide range of foods and drinks. They can be eaten fresh, frozen, or dried, and are commonly used in baked goods, smoothies, and salads. Strawberry shortcake, blueberry muffins, raspberry sorbet, and blackberry cobbler are just a few examples of the many delicious ways to enjoy berries.

In addition to their culinary uses, berries have been used for medicinal purposes for centuries. For example, cranberries are known to help prevent urinary tract infections, while elderberries have been shown to have antiviral properties and may help reduce the severity of cold and flu symptoms.

In conclusion, berries are a delicious and nutritious group of fruits that have many health benefits. They are a rich source of vitamins, minerals, and antioxidants, and are low in calories and high in fiber. Berries are a versatile ingredient in a wide range of foods and drinks and can be enjoyed in many different ways. Whether eaten fresh, frozen, or dried, berries are a delicious and healthy addition to any diet.

C. Stone fruits

Stone fruits, also known as drupes, are a group of fruits that have a hard stone or pit at their center. The stone surrounds a single seed, which is often eaten along with the fruit. Popular stone fruits include peaches, nectarines, apricots, plums, and cherries. Stone fruits are not only delicious but also have numerous health benefits, making them a popular choice for people looking to add more fruit to their diet.

Stone fruits are native to many different parts of the world, including Asia, Europe, and the Americas. They are grown on trees and are usually harvested by hand. Stone fruits are a rich source of vitamins, minerals, and antioxidants, and they are low in calories and high in fiber.

One of the key health benefits of stone fruits is their high content of vitamin C and vitamin A, both of which are important for immune system health and maintaining healthy skin and eyes. They are also a good source of dietary fiber, which can help regulate digestion and reduce the risk of heart disease and type 2 diabetes.

In addition to their nutritional value, stone fruits have many culinary uses. They can be eaten fresh or cooked, and are commonly used in baked goods, jams, and jellies. Peach cobbler, cherry pie, and plum jam are just a few examples of the many delicious ways to enjoy stone fruits.

Stone fruits have also been used for medicinal purposes for centuries. For example, apricots have been used in traditional Chinese medicine to treat respiratory ailments, while cherries have been shown to have anti-inflammatory properties and may help reduce muscle soreness and improve sleep.

In conclusion, stone fruits are a delicious and nutritious group of fruits that have many health benefits. They are a rich source of vitamins, minerals, and antioxidants, and are low in calories and high in fiber. Stone fruits are a versatile ingredient in a wide range of foods and drinks and can be enjoyed in many different ways. Whether eaten fresh or cooked, stone fruits are a delicious and healthy addition to any diet.

D. Tropical fruits

Tropical fruits are a group of fruits that are native to or commonly grown in tropical regions around the world, such as Southeast Asia, South America, and the Caribbean. These fruits are known for their bright colors, unique flavors, and numerous health benefits. Popular tropical fruits include mangoes, pineapples, papayas, bananas, and guavas. Tropical fruits are a rich source of vitamins, minerals, and antioxidants, and are often high in fiber. For example, mangoes are high in vitamin C, vitamin A, and dietary fiber, while papayas are a rich source of vitamin C, vitamin A, and potassium. Pineapples are high in vitamin C and manganese, while bananas are a good source of vitamin C, vitamin B6, and potassium.

In addition to their nutritional value, tropical fruits have many culinary uses. They can be eaten fresh or cooked, and are commonly used in smoothies, juices, and desserts. Mango salsa, pineapple upside-down cake, and banana bread are just a few examples of the many delicious ways to enjoy tropical fruits.

Tropical fruits also have a long history of use in traditional medicine. For example, guava leaves have been used in traditional medicine to treat diarrhea and fever, while papayas have been used to aid digestion and relieve constipation.

One of the challenges of tropical fruits is that they can be difficult to transport and store due to their delicate nature. However, many tropical fruits are now available in supermarkets and specialty stores year-round thanks to advances in technology and transportation.

In conclusion, tropical fruits are a delicious and nutritious group of fruits that have many health benefits. They are a rich source of vitamins, minerals, and antioxidants, and are often high in fiber. Tropical fruits are a versatile ingredient in a wide range of foods and drinks and can be enjoyed in many different ways. Whether eaten fresh or cooked, tropical fruits are a delicious and healthy addition to any diet.

E. Exotic fruits

Exotic fruits are a group of fruits that are not commonly found in traditional Western diets but are increasingly becoming more popular due to their unique flavors, nutritional value, and potential health benefits. These fruits are often sourced from tropical regions around the world and include fruits such as dragon fruit, rambutan, durian, and jackfruit.

Exotic fruits are a rich source of vitamins, minerals, and antioxidants. For example, dragon fruit is high in vitamin C and fiber, while rambutan is a good source of vitamin C, iron, and potassium. Durian is a good source of vitamin C, thiamin, and potassium, while jackfruit is high in fiber and vitamin C.

In addition to their nutritional value, exotic fruits have many culinary uses. They can be eaten fresh or cooked and are often used in smoothies, juices, and desserts. Dragon fruit sorbet, rambutan salad, durian smoothies, and jackfruit curry are just a few examples of the many delicious ways to enjoy exotic fruits.

Exotic fruits are also increasingly being studied for their potential health benefits. For example, durian has been shown to have anti-inflammatory and antioxidant properties, while jackfruit has been shown to have cholesterol-lowering effects.

One of the challenges of exotic fruits is that they can be difficult to find and may be more expensive than traditional fruits. However, many exotic fruits are now more widely available in specialty stores and supermarkets, and some can even be grown in certain regions with favorable climates.

In conclusion, exotic fruits are a delicious and nutritious group of fruits that have many health benefits. They are a rich source of vitamins, minerals, and antioxidants, and are often high in fiber. Exotic fruits are a versatile ingredient in a wide range of foods and drinks and can be enjoyed in many different ways. Whether eaten fresh or cooked, exotic fruits are a delicious and healthy addition to any diet.

F. Seasonal fruits

Seasonal fruits are a group of fruits that are only available during certain times of the year, usually when they are at the peak of their freshness and flavor. These fruits are often grown locally and are harvested and sold during their specific season. Examples of seasonal fruits include strawberries in the summer, apples in the fall, and oranges in the winter. Seasonal fruits are a great way to enjoy the freshest and most flavorful produce. When fruits are in season, they are at their peak ripeness and are usually harvested and sold locally. This means that they do not need to be transported long distances, and they can be sold at a lower cost than when they are out of season. Additionally, when fruits are in season, they are often more abundant, making them more widely available and easier to find.

Eating seasonal fruits is not only a great way to enjoy the freshest produce, but it can also have many health benefits. Seasonal fruits are often higher in nutrients than out-of-season fruits because they are grown in their natural environment and are allowed to ripen fully. Additionally, because they are usually grown locally, they are not exposed to the same level of pesticides and chemicals as fruits that are shipped long distances. Eating seasonal fruits can also have environmental benefits. When fruits are grown locally and consumed in season, they require less transportation, which means they have a lower carbon footprint. Additionally, buying seasonal fruits from local farmers can support the local economy and promote sustainable farming practices.

In conclusion, seasonal fruits are a great way to enjoy the freshest and most flavorful produce while also promoting good health and sustainable farming practices. By eating fruits that are in season, you can enjoy a wide variety of delicious and nutritious produce throughout the year, while also supporting your local farmers and reducing your carbon footprint.

G. Nutritious fruits

Fruits are an important component of a healthy and balanced diet. They are rich in vitamins, minerals, fiber, and antioxidants that are essential for optimal health. Some fruits are especially nutrient-dense and provide an array of health benefits beyond just basic nutrition.

Here are some of the most nutritious fruits:

1. Blueberries: Blueberries are a rich source of antioxidants and phytochemicals that can help reduce inflammation and improve brain function.
2. Avocado: Although technically a fruit, avocados are often considered a healthy fat. They are rich in heart-healthy monounsaturated fats and fiber, and also provide a variety of vitamins and minerals.
3. Pomegranate: Pomegranates are a rich source of antioxidants and polyphenols, which have been shown to have anti-inflammatory and anti-cancer properties.
4. Kiwi: Kiwi is a great source of vitamin C, fiber, and potassium. It also contains actinidin, an enzyme that can aid in digestion.
5. Mango: Mangoes are rich in vitamins A and C, fiber, and antioxidants. They have been shown to have anti-inflammatory properties and may also have beneficial effects on heart health.
6. Papaya: Papaya is a rich source of vitamins A and C, as well as an enzyme called papain, which can aid in digestion and may also have anti-inflammatory effects.
7. Guava: Guava is a great source of vitamin C and fiber, and also contains antioxidants that can help reduce inflammation.
8. Watermelon: Watermelon is a great source of hydration and is also rich in vitamin C, lycopene, and potassium. It may also have beneficial effects on heart health.

Incorporating a variety of nutritious fruits into your diet can provide numerous health benefits. Not only do they provide essential vitamins and minerals, but they also contain antioxidants and phytochemicals that can help reduce inflammation and improve overall health. Adding these fruits to your diet can be as simple as snacking on them throughout the day, adding them to smoothies or salads, or using them as a natural sweetener in baked goods.

IV. Health Benefits of Fruits

A. Fruits and their impact on disease prevention

Fruits are an essential part of a healthy diet and have been shown to have a positive impact on disease prevention. Fruits are naturally low in calories, high in fiber, and rich in vitamins and minerals, which can help prevent a variety of chronic diseases. Here are some ways that fruits can help prevent disease:

1. Heart Disease: Eating a diet rich in fruits has been linked to a lower risk of heart disease. Fruits are low in saturated fats and high in fiber, which can help lower cholesterol levels and reduce the risk of heart disease.

2. Cancer: Fruits contain a variety of phytochemicals, including antioxidants, which have been shown to have anti-cancer properties. Eating a diet rich in fruits, especially those with dark or bright colors, can help reduce the risk of certain types of cancer, including lung, breast, and colon cancer.

3. Type 2 Diabetes: Fruits are a great source of fiber, which can help regulate blood sugar levels and prevent insulin resistance. Eating a diet rich in fruits, especially those with a low glycemic index, can help reduce the risk of developing type 2 diabetes.

4. Obesity: Fruits are low in calories and high in fiber, which can help promote feelings of fullness and reduce overall calorie intake. Eating a diet rich in fruits can help promote weight loss and reduce the risk of obesity.

5. Digestive Health: Fruits are a great source of fiber, which can help promote digestive health and prevent constipation. Eating a

diet rich in fruits can help reduce the risk of digestive disorders, including diverticulitis and irritable bowel syndrome.

In conclusion, fruits are an essential part of a healthy diet and have been shown to have a positive impact on disease prevention. Eating a variety of fruits can provide numerous health benefits and help reduce the risk of chronic diseases, including heart disease, cancer, type 2 diabetes, obesity, and digestive disorders. Incorporating fruits into your diet can be as simple as snacking on them throughout the day, adding them to smoothies or salads, or using them as a natural sweetener in baked goods.

B. Nutrients found in fruits and their health benefits

Fruits are not only delicious and refreshing, but they also provide a plethora of essential nutrients that are important for our health. Here are some of the key nutrients found in fruits and their health benefits:

1. Vitamins: Fruits are rich in a variety of vitamins, including vitamins A, C, and E. Vitamin A is important for maintaining healthy skin and vision, while vitamin C is essential for a strong immune system and healthy skin. Vitamin E is a powerful antioxidant that helps protect our cells from damage caused by free radicals.

2. Minerals: Fruits are also a good source of minerals, including potassium, magnesium, and calcium. Potassium is important for maintaining healthy blood pressure and heart function, while magnesium is important for maintaining healthy bones and muscles. Calcium is essential for strong bones and teeth.

3. Fiber: Fruits are a great source of fiber, which is important for maintaining healthy digestion and preventing constipation. Fiber also helps reduce cholesterol levels and can lower the risk of heart disease and type 2 diabetes.

4. Antioxidants: Fruits are rich in antioxidants, which help protect our cells from damage caused by free radicals. Antioxidants are important for preventing chronic diseases such as cancer, heart disease, and Alzheimer's disease.

5. Water: Fruits are high in water content, which helps keep us hydrated and promotes healthy skin and digestion.

In addition to these key nutrients, fruits also provide a variety of other health benefits. For example, some fruits, such as blueberries and cherries, contain compounds that have been shown to reduce inflammation and improve brain function. Other fruits, such as kiwi and papaya, contain enzymes that aid in digestion and can help reduce bloating. Incorporating a variety of fruits into your diet is an easy way to ensure that you are getting a wide range of essential nutrients and reaping the health benefits that come with them. Try adding fruits to your meals, snacking on them throughout the day, or blending them into smoothies for a quick and delicious nutrient boost.

C. The role of fruits in maintaining a healthy weight

Fruits are an essential part of a healthy diet, and they play a vital role in maintaining a healthy weight. With their high fiber and low calorie content, fruits are the perfect food to help you feel full and satisfied while also providing important nutrients that your body needs. In this article, we will explore the many ways in which fruits can help you maintain a healthy weight.

1. Fruits are low in calories

One of the main reasons why fruits are so beneficial for weight management is that they are low in calories. Most fruits are made up of mostly water and fiber, which means that they contain very few calories compared to other foods. For example, a medium-sized apple contains only about 95 calories, while a medium-sized banana has around 105 calories. By replacing higher calorie snacks with fruits, you can reduce your overall calorie intake and promote weight loss.

2. Fruits are high in fiber

Fiber is a type of carbohydrate that cannot be digested by the body, and it plays a crucial role in maintaining a healthy weight. When you eat fiber-rich foods, such as fruits, you feel fuller for longer periods, which means you are less likely to overeat. Fiber also slows down the absorption of carbohydrates in the body, which can help to stabilize blood sugar levels and reduce cravings for sugary foods.

3. Fruits are nutrient-dense

Fruits are not only low in calories and high in fiber, but they are also packed with essential vitamins and minerals. By incorporating a variety of fruits into your diet, you can ensure that your body is getting all the nutrients it needs to function properly. This can be especially important for weight management because when your body is getting the nutrients it needs, you are less likely to crave unhealthy foods that can lead to weight gain.

4. Fruits can help prevent chronic diseases

Eating a diet that is rich in fruits has been linked to a lower risk of chronic diseases, such as heart disease, diabetes, and certain types of cancer. By maintaining a healthy weight, you can reduce your risk of developing these diseases, and incorporating fruits into your diet is an excellent way to do this. Fruits are also rich in antioxidants, which can help to reduce inflammation in the body and promote overall health.

In conclusion, fruits are an essential part of a healthy diet, and they play a vital role in maintaining a healthy weight. By incorporating a variety of fruits into your diet, you can benefit from their low calorie, high fiber, and nutrient-dense properties. Additionally, by maintaining a healthy weight through a diet rich in fruits and vegetables, you can reduce

D. Fruits and their impact on brain function

Fruits are not only delicious and nutritious, but they also play a critical role in maintaining brain function. The brain is one of the most important organs in the body, and it requires proper nutrition to function correctly. In this article, we will explore the impact of fruits on brain function and why they should be an essential part of your diet.

1. Fruits are rich in antioxidants

Fruits are a rich source of antioxidants, which play a crucial role in protecting the brain from damage caused by free radicals. Free radicals are unstable molecules that can damage cells and lead to cognitive decline. Antioxidants help to neutralize free radicals, reducing the risk of damage to brain cells.

2. Fruits are rich in vitamins and minerals

Fruits are also rich in essential vitamins and minerals that are important for brain function. For example, vitamin C, found in citrus fruits, is an antioxidant that helps protect the brain from damage. Folate, found in leafy green vegetables and citrus fruits, is essential for brain function and has been linked to a lower risk of cognitive decline.

3. Fruits can improve cognitive function

Studies have shown that eating fruits can improve cognitive function, including memory, attention, and processing speed. The antioxidants and other nutrients found in fruits can help to protect the brain from damage and reduce inflammation, which can improve cognitive function.

4. Fruits can reduce the risk of dementia

Dementia is a condition characterized by a decline in cognitive function that can interfere with daily life. Studies have shown that eating a diet rich in fruits can reduce the risk of dementia. One study found that people who ate a diet rich in fruits and vegetables had a 30% lower risk of developing dementia compared to those who ate a diet low in fruits and vegetables.

5.   Fruits can improve mood

Fruits can also improve mood, which can impact brain function. Studies have shown that people who eat a diet rich in fruits and vegetables are less likely to experience symptoms of depression and anxiety. The nutrients found in fruits, such as vitamin C and folate, can help to regulate mood and reduce stress.

In conclusion, fruits are an essential part of a healthy diet, and they play a critical role in maintaining brain function. The antioxidants, vitamins, and minerals found in fruits can help protect the brain from damage, improve cognitive function, reduce the risk of dementia, and improve mood. By incorporating a variety of fruits into your diet, you can benefit from their many health benefits and support optimal brain function.

E. Fruits and their impact on skin health

Fruits are not only delicious, but they are also packed with essential nutrients that can have a positive impact on skin health. The skin is the largest organ in the body, and it requires proper nutrition to look and feel its best. In this article, we will explore the impact of fruits on skin health and why they should be an essential part of your diet.

1. Fruits are rich in antioxidants

Fruits are a rich source of antioxidants, which play a critical role in protecting the skin from damage caused by free radicals. Free radicals are unstable molecules that can damage cells and lead to premature aging, wrinkles, and other skin damage. Antioxidants help to neutralize free radicals, reducing the risk of damage to skin cells.

2. Fruits are rich in vitamins and minerals

Fruits are also rich in essential vitamins and minerals that are important for skin health. For example, vitamin C, found in citrus fruits, is an antioxidant that helps to protect the skin from damage caused by the sun and pollution. Vitamin A, found in sweet potatoes and carrots, is important for maintaining healthy skin and has been shown to reduce the risk of acne.

3. Fruits can improve skin hydration

Eating fruits can also improve skin hydration, which is essential for maintaining healthy skin. Fruits such as watermelon, strawberries, and cucumbers have a high water content, which can help to hydrate the skin from the inside out. Proper hydration can help to reduce the appearance of fine lines and wrinkles and give the skin a more youthful appearance.

4. Fruits can reduce inflammation

Inflammation is a common cause of skin damage, and eating fruits can help to reduce inflammation in the body. Fruits such as berries, cherries, and grapes are rich in anthocyanins, which have been shown to reduce inflammation and improve skin health. Reducing inflammation can help to improve the overall appearance of the skin and reduce the risk of skin damage.

5. Fruits can promote collagen production

Collagen is a protein that is essential for healthy skin, and eating fruits can help to promote collagen production. Fruits such as kiwi, papaya, and mango are rich in vitamin C, which is essential for collagen production. Collagen can help to improve skin elasticity and reduce the appearance of wrinkles and fine lines.

In conclusion, fruits are an essential part of a healthy diet, and they play a critical role in maintaining healthy skin. The antioxidants, vitamins, and minerals found in fruits can help to protect the skin from damage, improve hydration, reduce inflammation, and promote collagen production. By incorporating a variety of fruits into your diet, you can benefit from their many health benefits and support optimal skin health.

V. Fruits and Disease Prevention

A. Fruits and their impact on cancer

Fruits are not only delicious, but they are also packed with essential nutrients that can have a positive impact on cancer prevention and treatment. Cancer is a complex disease that can be influenced by many factors, including diet. In this article, we will explore the impact of fruits on cancer and why they should be an essential part of your diet.

1. Fruits are rich in antioxidants

Fruits are a rich source of antioxidants, which play a critical role in protecting the body from damage caused by free radicals. Free radicals are unstable molecules that can damage cells and lead to cancer. Antioxidants help to neutralize free radicals, reducing the risk of damage to cells and lowering the risk of cancer.

2. Fruits are rich in fiber

Fruits are also rich in fiber, which can help to reduce the risk of cancer. Fiber helps to promote bowel regularity, which can reduce the risk of colon cancer. Fiber also helps to reduce inflammation, which can lower the risk of other types of cancer.

3. Fruits can reduce inflammation

Inflammation is a common cause of cancer, and eating fruits can help to reduce inflammation in the body. Fruits such as berries, cherries, and grapes are rich in anthocyanins, which have been shown to reduce inflammation and lower the risk of cancer. Reducing inflammation can help to improve overall health and reduce the risk of cancer.

4. Fruits can promote detoxification

Eating fruits can also help to promote detoxification, which can help to lower the risk of cancer. Fruits such as berries, citrus fruits, and apples are rich in antioxidants and other nutrients that can help to support the body's natural detoxification processes.

5.   Fruits can improve immune function

The immune system plays a critical role in fighting cancer, and eating fruits can help to improve immune function. Fruits such as citrus fruits, kiwi, and berries are rich in vitamin C, which is essential for immune function. Eating a diet rich in fruits can help to support immune function and lower the risk of cancer.

In conclusion, fruits are an essential part of a healthy diet, and they play a critical role in preventing and treating cancer. The antioxidants, fiber, anti-inflammatory compounds, and other nutrients found in fruits can help to protect the body from damage, improve immune function, and lower the risk of cancer. By incorporating a variety of fruits into your diet, you can benefit from their many health benefits and support optimal health.

B. Fruits and their impact on heart disease

Fruits are not only delicious, but they are also packed with essential nutrients that can have a positive impact on heart health. Heart disease is a leading cause of death worldwide, and diet plays a critical role in its prevention and treatment. In this article, we will explore the impact of fruits on heart disease and why they should be an essential part of your diet.

1. Fruits are rich in fiber

Fruits are a rich source of fiber, which can help to reduce the risk of heart disease. Fiber helps to lower cholesterol levels, reduce blood pressure, and promote bowel regularity. All of these factors can help to lower the risk of heart disease.

2. Fruits are rich in antioxidants

Fruits are also a rich source of antioxidants, which can help to protect the heart from damage caused by free radicals. Free radicals are unstable molecules that can damage cells and contribute to the development of heart disease. Antioxidants help to neutralize free radicals, reducing the risk of damage to cells and lowering the risk of heart disease.

3. Fruits can help to control blood sugar

High blood sugar levels can contribute to the development of heart disease, and eating fruits can help to control blood sugar levels. Fruits such as berries, apples, and citrus fruits have a low glycemic index, which means they release sugar into the bloodstream slowly. This can help to control blood sugar levels and lower the risk of heart disease.

4. Fruits can reduce inflammation

Inflammation is a common cause of heart disease, and eating fruits can help to reduce inflammation in the body. Fruits such as berries, cherries, and grapes are rich in anthocyanins, which have been shown to reduce inflammation and lower the risk of heart disease. Reducing inflammation can help to improve overall health and lower the risk of heart disease.

5.   Fruits can help to maintain a healthy weight

Maintaining a healthy weight is important for heart health, and eating fruits can help to support weight loss and weight management. Fruits are low in calories and high in fiber, which can help to promote feelings of fullness and reduce overall calorie intake. This can help to support weight loss and maintain a healthy weight, which can lower the risk of heart disease.

In conclusion, fruits are an essential part of a heart-healthy diet, and they play a critical role in preventing and treating heart disease. The fiber, antioxidants, anti-inflammatory compounds, and other nutrients found in fruits can help to lower cholesterol levels, control blood sugar, reduce inflammation, support weight loss, and promote overall heart health. By incorporating a variety of fruits into your diet, you can benefit from their many health benefits and support optimal heart health.

C. Fruits and their impact on diabetes

Fruits are a delicious and nutritious addition to any diet, but for those living with diabetes, the impact of fruits on blood sugar levels can be a concern. However, fruits are an essential source of essential nutrients that can have a positive impact on diabetes management. In this article, we will explore the impact of fruits on diabetes and why they should be an essential part of a diabetes-friendly diet.

1. Fruits are low in glycemic index

Fruits are low on the glycemic index, which means they release sugar into the bloodstream slowly, reducing the risk of spikes in blood sugar levels. This can be particularly beneficial for those with diabetes, as it can help to control blood sugar levels.

2. Fruits are a good source of fiber

Fruits are a rich source of dietary fiber, which can help to slow down the absorption of sugar into the bloodstream, further supporting blood sugar control. Fiber can also help to improve bowel regularity and reduce the risk of heart disease.

3. Fruits are rich in antioxidants

Fruits are also rich in antioxidants, which can help to protect against the damage caused by free radicals and lower the risk of complications associated with diabetes. Antioxidants help to neutralize free radicals, reducing the risk of damage to cells and promoting overall health.

4. Fruits can reduce the risk of complications

Eating fruits regularly can also help to reduce the risk of complications associated with diabetes, including heart disease and nerve damage. The fiber, antioxidants, and other essential nutrients found in fruits can help to improve overall health and support diabetes management.

5. Fruits can help to maintain a healthy weight

Maintaining a healthy weight is important for diabetes management, and eating fruits can help to support weight loss and weight management. Fruits are low in calories and high in fiber, which can help to promote feelings of fullness and reduce overall calorie intake. This can help to support weight loss and maintain a healthy weight, which can lower the risk of complications associated with diabetes.

In conclusion, fruits are an essential part of a diabetes-friendly diet, and they play a critical role in diabetes management. The low glycemic index, fiber, antioxidants, and other essential nutrients found in fruits can help to support blood sugar control, reduce the risk of complications, promote overall health, and support weight management. By incorporating a variety of fruits into your diet, you can benefit from their many health benefits and support optimal diabetes management.

D. Fruits and their impact on digestive health

Fruits are an essential part of a healthy diet, and they can have a positive impact on digestive health. Digestive health is critical for overall health and wellbeing, and diet plays a critical role in maintaining optimal digestive function. In this article, we will explore the impact of fruits on digestive health and why they should be an essential part of your diet.

1. Fruits are a rich source of dietary fiber

Fruits are a rich source of dietary fiber, which can help to promote digestive health. Fiber helps to promote bowel regularity, prevent constipation, and reduce the risk of digestive disorders such as diverticulitis and colon cancer.

2. Fruits can improve nutrient absorption

Fruits are also rich in essential nutrients such as vitamins and minerals that are critical for optimal digestive function. By consuming fruits, you can ensure that your body has the necessary nutrients to support digestive health, and you can improve nutrient absorption.

3. Fruits can support the growth of healthy gut bacteria

Fruits contain prebiotic fiber, which can support the growth of healthy gut bacteria. Healthy gut bacteria are critical for optimal digestive function, and they play a critical role in supporting overall health and wellbeing.

4. Fruits can reduce inflammation

Inflammation is a common cause of digestive disorders, and consuming fruits can help to reduce inflammation in the body. Fruits such as berries, cherries, and grapes are rich in antioxidants and anti-inflammatory compounds that can help to reduce inflammation and support digestive health.

5. Fruits can support weight management

Maintaining a healthy weight is important for digestive health, and consuming fruits can help to support weight management. Fruits are low in calories and high in fiber, which can help to promote feelings of fullness and reduce overall calorie intake. This can help to support weight loss and maintain a healthy weight, which can promote digestive health. In conclusion, fruits are an essential part of a healthy diet, and they can have a positive impact on digestive health. The fiber, essential nutrients, prebiotic fiber, anti-inflammatory compounds, and other essential nutrients found in fruits can help to promote bowel regularity, improve nutrient absorption, support the growth of healthy gut bacteria, reduce inflammation, and support weight management. By incorporating a variety of fruits into your diet, you can benefit from their many health benefits and support optimal digestive health.

E. Fruits and their impact on respiratory health

Fruits are an essential part of a healthy diet, and they can have a positive impact on respiratory health. Respiratory health is critical for overall health and wellbeing, and diet plays a critical role in maintaining optimal respiratory function. In this article, we will explore the impact of fruits on respiratory health and why they should be an essential part of your diet.

1. Fruits are a rich source of antioxidants

Fruits are a rich source of antioxidants, which can help to protect the respiratory system from oxidative stress. Oxidative stress is a common cause of respiratory disorders, and consuming fruits can help to reduce oxidative stress and promote respiratory health.

2. Fruits can reduce inflammation

Inflammation is a common cause of respiratory disorders, and consuming fruits can help to reduce inflammation in the body. Fruits such as berries, cherries, and grapes are rich in anti-inflammatory compounds that can help to reduce inflammation and support respiratory health.

3. Fruits can support lung function

Fruits are also rich in essential nutrients such as vitamins A and C, which can support lung function. Vitamin A is essential for the development of healthy lung tissue, while vitamin C can help to reduce the risk of respiratory infections and promote overall respiratory health.

4. Fruits can improve immune function

The immune system plays a critical role in protecting the respiratory system from infections and other disorders. Fruits are rich in essential nutrients such as vitamins A and C, as well as other immune-supporting compounds, which can help to improve immune function and support respiratory health.

5. Fruits can support overall health

Maintaining overall health is critical for respiratory health, and consuming fruits can help to support overall health and wellbeing. Fruits are low in calories and high in essential nutrients, fiber, and other compounds that can promote overall health and reduce the risk of chronic diseases.

In conclusion, fruits are an essential part of a healthy diet, and they can have a positive impact on respiratory health. The antioxidants, anti-inflammatory compounds, essential nutrients, and immune-supporting compounds found in fruits can help to protect the respiratory system from oxidative stress and inflammation, support lung function, improve immune function, and support overall health and wellbeing. By incorporating a variety of fruits into your diet, you can benefit from their many health benefits and support optimal respiratory health.

VI. Incorporating Fruits into your Diet

A. How to choose the right fruits

Choosing the right fruits can be a daunting task, especially with so many options available in the market. However, it's essential to make the right choices when selecting fruits as they form an integral part of a healthy diet. In this article, we will explore some tips on how to choose the right fruits.

1. Seasonal fruits

Choosing fruits that are in season is the best way to ensure that they are fresh and packed with essential nutrients. Seasonal fruits are also likely to be more affordable and taste better than fruits that are out of season. Moreover, buying seasonal fruits helps to support local farmers and reduces the carbon footprint associated with transporting fruits from faraway places.

2. Choose ripe fruits

When choosing fruits, it's essential to look for those that are ripe but not overripe. Overripe fruits may have a mushy texture and may not taste good. On the other hand, unripe fruits may lack flavor and essential nutrients. To check if a fruit is ripe, gently press it with your fingers. If it yields to pressure, it's likely to be ripe.

3. Color

Fruits come in different colors, and each color represents a unique set of nutrients. For instance, oranges and mangoes are rich in vitamin C, while dark-colored berries are rich in antioxidants. When choosing fruits, consider the color to ensure that you get a variety of nutrients in your diet.

4. Check for bruises and cuts

It's essential to examine fruits carefully before purchasing to ensure that they are free from bruises and cuts. Damaged fruits are likely to spoil quickly, and they may harbor harmful bacteria, which can cause foodborne illnesses.

5.   Organic vs. conventionally grown fruits

Organic fruits are grown without the use of synthetic fertilizers, pesticides, and herbicides. They are considered healthier and more environmentally friendly than conventionally grown fruits. However, organic fruits may be more expensive than conventionally grown fruits. If you're on a budget, you can choose conventionally grown fruits, but be sure to wash them thoroughly to remove any pesticide residues.

In conclusion, choosing the right fruits is essential for maintaining optimal health and wellbeing. When selecting fruits, consider the season, ripeness, color, condition, and whether they are organic or conventionally grown. By making the right choices, you can enjoy a variety of fruits that are packed with essential nutrients and delicious flavors.

B. How to prepare and store fruits

Fruits are an essential part of a healthy diet, and they should be prepared and stored properly to retain their nutrients and flavors. In this article, we will explore some tips on how to prepare and store fruits.

1. Washing fruits

Before consuming or storing fruits, it's essential to wash them thoroughly. Washing removes dirt, bacteria, and pesticides, which can cause foodborne illnesses. To wash fruits, place them in a colander and rinse them under running water. For delicate fruits like berries, rinse them gently and pat them dry with a paper towel.

2. Peeling fruits

Some fruits like bananas and oranges can be consumed without peeling, while others like apples and pears need to be peeled. Peeling fruits removes the skin, which may contain pesticide residues and dirt. To peel fruits, use a sharp knife or a peeler and remove the skin in a circular motion.

3. Cutting fruits

Cutting fruits into smaller pieces makes them easier to consume and cook. To cut fruits, use a sharp knife and cut them into even-sized pieces. For fruits like apples and pears, remove the core and seeds before cutting.

4. Storing fruits

Fruits should be stored properly to retain their flavor and nutrients. Different fruits have different storage requirements. Some fruits like bananas and apples can be stored at room temperature, while others like berries and grapes need to be refrigerated.

a. Room temperature storage

Fruits that can be stored at room temperature include bananas, avocados, and citrus fruits. Store these fruits in a cool, dry place away from direct sunlight.

b. Refrigerator storage

Fruits that need to be refrigerated include berries, grapes, and melons. Store these fruits in the crisper drawer of the refrigerator to maintain their freshness.

c. Freezer storage

Some fruits can be frozen for later use. Freezing fruits preserves their nutrients and flavor. To freeze fruits, wash and cut them into small pieces and place them in a freezer bag. Store the bag in the freezer for up to six months.

5. Avoid overripe fruits

Overripe fruits can spoil quickly and may contain harmful bacteria. It's essential to consume or use overripe fruits as soon as possible or discard them if they are spoiled.

In conclusion, preparing and storing fruits properly is essential for maintaining their flavor and nutrients. To prepare fruits, wash, peel, and cut them into smaller pieces. To store fruits, consider their storage requirements and store them in the appropriate place. By following these tips, you can enjoy fresh and nutritious fruits all year round.

C. Fruit-based recipes

Fruits are not only delicious, but they are also packed with essential vitamins and nutrients that are crucial for maintaining good health. Incorporating fruits into your diet can be done in many ways, including using them in recipes. Here are some delicious fruit-based recipes that you can try out:

1. Berry Smoothie Bowl: A smoothie bowl is an excellent way to start your day, and this one is filled with delicious berries. Blend together frozen berries, banana, almond milk, and honey until smooth. Pour the mixture into a bowl and top it with your favorite toppings such as sliced bananas, chia seeds, and granola.

2. Mango Salsa: Mango salsa is a perfect appetizer or side dish to accompany grilled chicken or fish. Combine diced mango, red onion, jalapeno, lime juice, and cilantro in a bowl. Serve with tortilla chips or as a topping for tacos.

3. Strawberry Salad: A refreshing salad that is perfect for a summer day. Toss together fresh spinach, sliced strawberries, crumbled feta cheese, and toasted almonds. Drizzle balsamic vinaigrette on top.

4. Grilled Pineapple: Grilled pineapple is a tasty dessert that is easy to make. Slice a fresh pineapple into rounds and brush them with honey. Grill the pineapple until it's lightly charred, and serve it with a dollop of whipped cream or vanilla ice cream.

5. Banana Bread: Banana bread is a classic recipe that is easy to make and perfect for using up ripe bananas. Mash ripe bananas and mix them with flour, sugar, baking powder, and eggs. Pour the mixture into a loaf pan and bake until golden brown.

6. Fruit Pizza: Fruit pizza is a fun and colorful dessert that is sure to impress. Use a sugar cookie dough for the crust and top it with

cream cheese frosting. Arrange sliced fruits such as strawberries, kiwis, and blueberries on top.

7.   Apple Cinnamon Oatmeal: A warm and comforting breakfast that is perfect for fall. Cook oats in water or milk and add chopped apples, cinnamon, and brown sugar. Top it with chopped nuts and a drizzle of honey.

In conclusion, fruits are a versatile ingredient that can be used in many different recipes. Try out these fruit-based recipes to add some variety to your diet and enjoy their delicious flavors.

D. Incorporating fruits into your daily routine

Incorporating fruits into your daily routine is a great way to improve your overall health and well-being. Fruits are packed with essential vitamins, minerals, and fiber that can help to reduce the risk of chronic diseases and promote good health. Here are some tips for incorporating fruits into your daily routine:

1. Start your day with a fruit-based breakfast: A fruit-based breakfast is a great way to kickstart your day. You can make a smoothie bowl, oatmeal with chopped fruits, or a fruit salad with yogurt and granola.

2. Snack on fruits: Snacking on fruits instead of processed snacks is an excellent way to curb your cravings and get some essential nutrients. You can slice up some apples, pears, or bananas and dip them in almond butter or hummus.

3. Add fruits to your lunch: Adding fruits to your lunch can help to balance out your meal and make it more nutritious. You can add sliced fruits to your salad, make a sandwich with avocado and sliced fruit, or have a fruit-based side dish.

4. Use fruits in your cooking: Fruits can be a great addition to your cooking, and they can add a natural sweetness to your dishes. You can add diced apples to your oatmeal or use mashed bananas in your baking recipes.

5. Make fruit-infused water: Drinking enough water is crucial for good health, and adding fruits to your water can make it more flavorful and enjoyable. You can add sliced citrus fruits, berries, or cucumbers to your water bottle.

6. Have a fruit-based dessert: Having a fruit-based dessert instead of sugary treats can satisfy your sweet tooth and provide you with

some essential nutrients. You can make a fruit salad, grilled fruit skewers, or a fruit-based sorbet.

In conclusion, incorporating fruits into your daily routine is a simple and effective way to improve your health and well-being. By following these tips, you can add more fruits to your diet and enjoy their delicious flavors and health benefits.

VII. Conclusion

A. Summary of the benefits of fruits

Fruits are an essential part of a healthy and balanced diet. They are packed with essential vitamins, minerals, and fiber that are crucial for good health. Here is a summary of the benefits of fruits:

1. Nutrient-rich: Fruits are loaded with essential vitamins and minerals that are vital for good health. They are particularly high in vitamin C, vitamin A, and potassium.
2. Fiber: Fruits are an excellent source of dietary fiber, which is essential for good digestion and preventing constipation.
3. Low in calories: Fruits are low in calories and high in water content, which makes them an ideal food for weight management.
4. Antioxidants: Fruits are rich in antioxidants, which help to protect the body against oxidative stress and reduce the risk of chronic diseases such as cancer, heart disease, and Alzheimer's disease.
5. Hydration: Fruits are high in water content, which makes them an ideal food for hydration. Eating fruits can help to keep you hydrated and prevent dehydration.
6. Immune system support: Fruits are rich in vitamin C, which is essential for a healthy immune system. Eating fruits can help to boost your immunity and reduce the risk of infections.
7. Skin health: Fruits are high in antioxidants and vitamin C, which can help to improve the health of your skin. Eating fruits can

help to reduce the signs of aging and promote healthy, glowing skin.

8. Heart health: Fruits are low in saturated fats and high in fiber, which can help to reduce the risk of heart disease. Eating fruits can help to lower blood pressure, reduce inflammation, and improve cholesterol levels.

In conclusion, fruits are an essential part of a healthy and balanced diet. They are packed with essential nutrients and offer a range of health benefits. By incorporating fruits into your daily diet, you can improve your overall health and well-being.

B. Final thoughts on the importance of fruits

Fruits are an essential part of a healthy and balanced diet. They are packed with essential vitamins, minerals, and fiber that are crucial for good health. In this article, we have explored the many benefits of fruits, including their nutrient-rich properties, high fiber content, low calorie count, antioxidant properties, hydration benefits, immune system support, skin health benefits, and heart health benefits.

Incorporating fruits into your daily diet is a simple and effective way to improve your health and well-being. Whether you enjoy fruits as a snack, in your meals, or as a dessert, there are many ways to incorporate them into your daily routine. By choosing a variety of fruits and eating them regularly, you can reap the benefits of their nutrient-rich properties and improve your overall health.

It is also important to note that consuming fruits as a part of a balanced diet is not only beneficial for your physical health but also your mental health. Eating a balanced diet with fruits can help improve your mood, increase energy levels, and reduce stress levels.

In conclusion, fruits are a vital component of a healthy diet. They offer a wide range of health benefits and can help to reduce the risk of chronic diseases. By making fruits a regular part of your diet, you can improve your overall health and well-being, both physically and mentally. So, the next time you are making a grocery list, be sure to include a variety of fruits to reap their many benefits.

C. Call to action: Incorporating fruits into your diet

Incorporating fruits into your diet is a simple and effective way to improve your health and well-being. Fruits are packed with essential nutrients, fiber, and antioxidants that are crucial for good health. However, despite the many benefits of fruits, many people do not consume enough of them in their daily diet.

If you are looking to improve your health and well-being, incorporating fruits into your diet is a great place to start. Here are some tips on how to do so:

1. Set a goal: Set a goal to consume a certain number of servings of fruits each day. The American Heart Association recommends at least 4-5 servings of fruits per day.
2. Plan ahead: Plan ahead and make sure you have a variety of fruits available in your home. This will make it easier to incorporate them into your meals and snacks.
3. Try new fruits: Don't be afraid to try new fruits that you haven't tried before. You may be surprised by how much you enjoy them.
4. Mix it up: Mix up the way you consume fruits. Try eating them fresh, frozen, or canned. You can also add them to your smoothies or make fruit-based desserts.
5. Make it a habit: Incorporating fruits into your diet is not a one-time thing. Make it a habit by consuming them regularly.

Incorporating fruits into your diet is not only good for your health but can also be a fun and tasty way to explore new flavors and recipes. So, take action today and make it a goal to incorporate more fruits into your daily diet. Your body will thank you for it!

D. Future research on the health benefits of fruits.

Fruits have been shown to have numerous health benefits, including reducing the risk of chronic diseases, improving digestion, and promoting healthy skin. However, there is still much to be learned about the potential health benefits of fruits.

As research on the health benefits of fruits continues, here are some areas that future studies may explore:

1. The role of fruit in cancer prevention: There is evidence that consuming fruits may help to reduce the risk of certain types of cancer, such as breast, colon, and lung cancer. Future studies may explore the specific compounds in fruits that have anti-cancer properties and how they may work to prevent cancer.

2. The effects of fruit on brain health: There is some evidence that consuming fruits may improve cognitive function and reduce the risk of neurodegenerative diseases, such as Alzheimer's disease. Future studies may explore the specific compounds in fruits that are responsible for these effects and how they work in the brain.

3. The impact of fruit on gut microbiome: The gut microbiome plays a crucial role in overall health, and there is evidence that consuming fruits may promote a healthy gut microbiome. Future studies may explore the specific types of fruits that are most beneficial for the gut microbiome and how they work to promote gut health.

4. The effects of fruit on inflammation: Chronic inflammation is associated with a range of health problems, including heart disease and diabetes. There is some evidence that consuming fruits may help to reduce inflammation in the body. Future studies may explore the specific compounds in fruits that have

anti-inflammatory properties and how they work to reduce inflammation.

5. The impact of fruit on athletic performance: Fruits are a natural source of carbohydrates and can be an excellent source of energy for athletes. Future studies may explore the specific types of fruits that are most beneficial for athletic performance and how they may improve endurance and recovery.

In conclusion, while we know that fruits offer a range of health benefits, there is still much to be learned about their potential benefits. As research on the health benefits of fruits continues, we may discover new ways in which fruits can improve our health and well-being.